JUMAYEVA MADINA FAXRITDINOVNA

FREQUENCY OF OCCURRENCE AND RISK FACTORS FOR THE DEVELOPMENT OF CHRONIC KIDNEY DISEASE IN WOMEN OF FERTILE AGE

Monograph

© Jumayeva Madina Faxritdinovna
Frequency of occurrence and risk factors for the development of Chronic Kidney disease in women of fertile age
By: Jumayeva Madina Faxritdinovna
Edition: January '2025
Publisher:
Taemeer Publications LLC (Michigan, USA / Hyderabad, India)

© Jumayeva Madina Faxritdinovna

Book	:	Frequency of occurrence and risk factors for the development of Chronic Kidney disease in women of fertile age
Author	:	Jumayeva Madina Faxritdinovna
Publisher	:	Taemeer Publications
Year	:	'2025
Pages	:	60
Title Design	:	*Taemeer Web Design*

Jumayeva Madina Faxritdinovna

Fertil yoshidagi ayollarda surunkali buyrak kasalligi rivojlanishining paydo bo`lish darajasi va xavf omillari [text]/Jumayeva Madina Faxritdinovna

/Buxoro — 2024. — 60 b.

Jumayeva Madina Faxritdinovna – Buxoro Davlat Tibbiyot Instituti , Fakultet va Gospital terapiya kafedrasi assistenti

Taqrizchilar:

Abdullaev R.B.	-	TTA, Urganch filiali, ichki kasalliklar, reobiliotologiya va xalq tabobati professori, tibbiyot fanlari doktori
Yo`ldosheva D.H.	-	Buxoro davlat tibbiyot instituti, klinik farmakologiya kafedrasi dotsenti, tibbiyot fanlari doktori

Ushbu monografiyada fertil yoshdagi ayollarda surunkali buyrak kasalligi uchrash darajasi, tarqalishi, xavf omillari yo'nalishida olib borilgan ilmiy izlanishlar haqida bayon etiladi. Monografiyada keltirilgan surunkali buyrak kasalligining tug'ish yoshidagi ayollar orasida uchrash chastotasi, qaysi xavf omillari ko'proq sabab bo'lishi ravon tilda bayon etilgan va ko'plab muammolarga urg'u berilgan. Qo'llanmadan tibbiyot institutlari, ordinatorlar, magistrlar, nefrolog, reabilitolog va terapevtlar uchun muhim qo'llanma sifatida amaliyotda foydalanish mumkin.

Jumayeva Madina Faxritdinovna

Frequency of occurrence and risk factors for the development of chronic kidney disease in women of fertile age [text]/Jumayeva Madina Faxritdinovna

/Bukhara — 2024. — 60 p.

Jumayeva Madina Faxritdinovna - Bukhara State Medical Institute, Faculty and assistant of the Department of hospital therapy

Reviewers:

Abdullaev R.B. - TTA, Urgench branch, professor of Internal Medicine, reobiliotology and folk medicine, doctor of Medical Sciences

Yo`ldosheva D.H. - BSMI, Associate Professor of the Department of Clinical Pharmacology, doctor of Medical Sciences

This monograph describes the scientific research carried out in the direction of the incidence, prevalence, risk factors of chronic kidney disease in women of fertile age. The frequency of occurrence of chronic kidney disease among women of childbearing age listed in the monograph, which risk factors are the most likely cause, is stated in fluent language and emphasizes many problems. The manual can be used in practice as an important guide for medical institutes, interns, Masters, nephrologists, rehabilitologists and therapists.

Жумаева Мадина Фахритдиновна

Частота встречаемости и факторы риска развития хронической болезни почек у женщин фертильного возраста [текст]/ Жумаева Мадина Фахритдиновна /Бухара — 2024. — 60 с.

Жумаева Мадина Фахритдиновна - Бухарский государственный медицинский институт, преподаватель и ассистент кафедры госпитальной терапии

Рецензенты:

Абдуллаев Р.Б. - ТТА, Ургенчский филиал, профессор кафедры внутренних болезней, реобилиотологии и народной медицины, доктор медицинских наук

Юлдашева Д.Х. - БГМИ, доцент кафедра клинической фармакологии, доктор медицинских наук

В данной монографии описаны научные исследования, проведенные в направлении изучения заболеваемости, распространенности, факторов риска хронических заболеваний почек у женщин фертильного возраста. Перечисленная в монографии частота встречаемости хронических заболеваний почек среди женщин детородного возраста, факторы риска которых являются наиболее вероятной причиной, изложены доступным языком и подчеркивают многие проблемы. Руководство может быть использовано на практике в качестве важного руководства для медицинских институтов, интернов, магистров, нефрологов, реабилитологов и терапевтов.

CONTENT

LIST OF ABBREVIATIONS ……………………………………………...

INTRODUCTION ……………………………………………………………..

CHAPTER 1. THE CONCEPT OF CKD (LITERATURE REVIEW)………………

1.1. The question of the prevalence of chronic kidney disease ……………..

1.2. CKD risk factors are a medical and social problem………………………

1.3. Diagnostic criteria for chronic kidney disease………………………………

1.4. Modern strategies for the detection of chronic kidney disease……………

CHAPTER II. MATERIALS AND METHODS OF RESEARCH …………

2.1 RESEARCH MATERIALS ……………………………………………………………..

2.2 RESEARCH DESIGN………………………………………………………………………

2.3 RESEARCH METHODS ……………………………………………………………..

CHAPTER III. ANALYSIS OF THE RESULTS OF THE FREQUENCY STUDY THE INCIDENCE OF CHRONIC KIDNEY DISEASE AMONG WOMEN OF FERTILE AGE…………………………

3.1. The frequency of occurrence of non-traditional factors as a factor the risk of developing CKD………………………………

3.2. The value of microalbuminuria/proteinuria as a predictor diagnosis and risk factors for CKD…………………

3.3. Factors associated with microalbuminuria………….

CHAPTER IV. THE PROGNOSTIC VALUE OF MICROALBUMINURIA IN ASSESSING THE CONDITION OF OVERWEIGHT AND OBESE KIDNEYS

4.1 Assessment of risk factors associated with albuminuria affecting on the development of chronic kidney disease……………………………………

4.2. Optimization algorithm for the tactics of early detection of chronic kidney diseases and ways to prevent progression……………

Conclusion………………………………………………………

Practical recommendations..

List of literature ………………………………………………..

LIST OF ABBREVIATED WORDS

AH- arterial hypertension

RRT – renal replacement therapy

IHD - ischemic heart disease

BMI- body mass index

HDL- high density lipoproteins

LDL- low density lipoproteins

MAU-microalbuminuria

NSAIDs - nonsteroidal anti–inflammatory drugs

GFR – glomerular filtration rate

CVC -cardiovascular complications

RFP- rural family polyclinic

TG – triglyceride

TRF – terminal renal failure

CKD - chronic kidney disease

CND - chronic non-communicable diseases

CKD-EPI-Chronic Kidney Desease Epidemiology Collaboration Index

KDOQI - Kidney Disease Outcomes Quality Initiative

MDRD - Modification of Diet in Renal Disease

INTRODUCTION

Today, chronic kidney disease (CKD) is a general medical problem with deep socio – medical and economic consequences associated with its widespread prevalence among the population, disability, mortality due to the development of kidney failure and cardiovascular complications.

In recent years, there has been a steady increase in patients with chronic renal disease. It was found that chronic kidney disease is observed in 12-80% of the population in countries with different ethnic composition and economic development, signs of chronic kidney disease of stages C3-C5, which are most unfavorable in 5.9-8.1% of residents, and in Japan up to 18.7%.

At the global level, a number of scientific studies are currently being conducted to achieve high reliability and efficiency in improving the early diagnosis, treatment and prevention of chronic kidney disease. In this regard, there is a sufficient number of scientific papers on the close, direct relationship of risk factors for the formation and development of chronic renal pathology with the level of complications and mortality among patients.

In research and medical centers of various countries, research works are carried out in the chosen field of research, but the features of early diagnosis and prevention, the importance of risk factors for the development and progression of chronic kidney disease, the assessment of the relationship between weight gain and the development of this pathology, the development of early biomarkers for diagnosis and an algorithm for early detection of chronic kidney disease are still being studied.

In our republic today, one of the priorities is to develop ways to improve the health care system, early detection and prevention of widespread non-communicable diseases, including nephrological diseases. The action strategy for 5 priority areas of the Republic of Uzbekistan in 2017-2021 states that " ... one of the main tasks is to improve the convenience and quality of medical care, strengthen the material and technical base of medical institutions, further reform specialized and high-tech medical care, strengthen family health...". The current tasks that are waiting to be solved at this time are to reduce the growth of chronic kidney disease among the population, to determine the significance of risk factors for the development and progression of chronic kidney disease, to develop an algorithm for early detection of chronic kidney disease and an early urinary biomarker for determining

This dissertation survey to a certain extent serves to fulfill the tasks set by the President of the Republic of Uzbekistan PP-3846 of July 12, 2018"On measures to improve the efficiency of providing nephrological and hemodialysis care to the population of the Republic of Uzbekistan".

Compliance of the research with the priority directions of development of science and technology of the republic.

The dissertation work was carried out in accordance with the priority directions of the development of science and technology of the Republic of Uzbekistan VI. "Medicine and Pharmacology".

The degree of knowledge of the problem. Chronic kidney disease (CKD) occupies a special place among chronic non-communicable diseases, since it is widespread, is associated with a sharp deterioration in the quality of life, high mortality, and in the terminal stage leads to the need for expensive methods of replacement therapy – dialysis and kidney transplantation (Vasilyeva I. A. et al., 2013; Bikbaev B. T., 2014; Soibov R. I., 2015; AlexanderR. T. etal., 2012; QaseemA. etal., 2013).

An increase in interest in this problem arose at the beginning of the XXI century, when new data from epidemiological studies (JMA) appeared. etal.,2008; JamesM.T., 2010; AroraP. etal. 2013; GansevoortR. T. etal., 2013), showing a high incidence of renal impairment in the population, and when it became apparent that dialysis services worldwide were not coping with the ever-increasing influx of patients with end-stage renal failure (ESRD).

A particular danger of CKD is that it can cause no complaints for a long time that would prompt the patient to consult a doctor, which brings it even closer to such well-known chronic diseases as diabetes mellitus and arterial hypertension (Galushkin A. A. et al., 2013).

It should be borne in mind that the problem of CKD is not fetal. Most of the risk factors for the development and progression of CKD can be corrected, and timely nephroprotective therapy reduces the likelihood of ESRD by 25-50%, which emphasizes the importance of early detection of CKD, its primary and secondary prevention (Kutaryna I. M., 2013; Podzolkov V. I., 2018).

The conducted studies established the main criteria for the diagnosis of CKD, which include the presence of any clinical and laboratory markers of kidney damage, primarily increased albuminuria/proteinuria, persisting for at least 3 months, irreversible structural changes in the kidney, detected by radiation examination; a decrease in GFR to the level of <60 ml / min/1, 73m2 and persisting for 3 months or more (Sigitova O. N., 2008; Smirnov A.V. et al., 2012).

It was found that for the level of albuminuria in the urine during screening examinations, a one-time study is preferred, rather than a daily urine sample using a semi - quantitative method (test strips), more accurate, but also expensive quantitative methods that are intended for nephrological examination to verify the diagnosis (Nagaytseva S. S., 2013; ClandiaM.etal., 2016).

One of the most promising methods for diagnosing CKD is the monitoring of registers and medical electronic databases. It is necessary to create regional, national registers of patients with CKD, which requires additional organizational efforts and financial costs. Studies conducted in the UK found that automated screening of 10975 records revealed 492 cases of CKD with C3a-5 (GullermoG., 2015).

About 10% of the world's adult population suffers from CKD, including nearly 200 million women worldwide. The diagnosis is made in the presence of any chronic kidney damage, even if their function is not impaired. The progression of CKD does not always occur, but in many cases, the deterioration of kidney function is observed for several years or even months and leads to the need for dialysis. Although the prevalence of CKD in women is on average 14%, and in men 12%, women receive dialysis less often than men. In addition, women around the world are more likely to become kidney donors for transplantation than recipients. The reasons for this situation are social, economic, and educational.

Numerous studies conducted in different countries indicate that the search for an optimal strategy for early detection of CKD through targeted screening, multi-faceted surveys of populations at increased risk of its development is in demand.

Purpose of the study To determine the frequency of occurrence and to study the risk factors for the development of chronic kidney disease and to optimize the tactics of prevention of its progression.

Research objectives:

1. Analysis of the occurrence and level of diagnosis of CKD among women of childbearing age in outpatient settings.

2. Identification of the causes and risk factors for the development of chronic kidney disease in women of fertile age.

3. Determination of diagnostic values of early markers of kidney damage in the examined groups.

4. Development of an algorithm for early detection of chronic kidney disease and prevention of its progression.

The object of the study was 87 women of fertile age.

The subject of the study was biological materials (blood, urine) obtained from patients, statistical and questionnaire material.

Research methods. The dissertation work was carried out using clinical, biochemical, hematological and statistical methods of research.

The scientific novelty is as follows:

- the most significant risk factors for the formation and development of CKD in women of childbearing age were identified, risk ranges were determined, which make it possible to include this pathology in the risk group and conduct secondary prevention
- determination of microalbuminuria is an early predictor of the diagnosis of CKD and predicting its progression in overweight and obese individuals;
- the diagnostic value of microalbuminuria, which in outpatient settings allows early detection and diagnosis of CKD in patients of different risk groups, has been proven;

- developed an algorithm for diagnosis and prevention, including risk factors for CKD

The practical results of the study consist of the following:

- a special "Questionnaire for identifying CKD risk factors" for mass screening studies has been developed and put into practice;
- it is recommended to determine microalbuminuria for the early diagnosis of CKD in women of childbearing age, a risk group, during mass screening examinations that do not involve blood tests;
- approaches to the secondary prevention of this pathology are recommended, taking into account the early diagnosis and prognosis of CKD in patients at risk.

The reliability of the results of the study is justified by the use of certain approaches and methods, the methodological correspondence of the conducted studies, the sufficiency of the number of respondents and patients examined, the processing of the material by statistical methods of the study, as well as the comparison of the results of the study with foreign and domestic materials, the confirmation of the results and conclusions by the competent authorities.

Scientific and practical significance of the research results.

The scientific significance of the study results consists of determining microalbuminuria as an early predictor of CKD diagnosis and predicting this pathology in patients at risk, including those with overweight and obesity, in identifying the most significant risk factors for the development and progression of CKD, which allows for secondary prevention of this disease, and developing a computer program that allows quantifying the integral risk of CKD development in the examined patients.

The practical significance of the study lies in the fact that a system of early diagnosis through the definition of microalbuminuria and comparative analysis of clinical, anamnestic, laboratory aspects of the course of CKD and " Questionnaire for identifying CKD risk factors for mass screening studies in rural areas. Recommendations for the use of microalbuminuria in mass screening studies and approaches to secondary prevention of this pathology have improved the early diagnosis of CKD in high-risk individuals permanently residing in rural areas and reduced the cases of CKD progression among rural residents.

Approbation of the research results. The main results of the dissertation work were reported at a number of scientific and practical conferences, including the number of international conferences.

Based on the materials of the dissertation, 4 scientific papers were published.

Structure and scope of the dissertation. The dissertation consists of an introduction, a review of the literature, a chapter materials and methods, 2 chapters with the presentation and analysis of the results of their own research, conclusions, conclusions, and a list of references. The volume is 78 pages.

CHAPTER I. THE CONCEPT OF CKD (Literature review)

§ 1.1 Prevalence, risk factors, and organization of medical care for chronic kidney disease

The development of clinical medicine in recent years allows to preserve the life, working capacity and social activity of patients, as well as to improve their quality of life. But it is not always possible to carry out timely diagnosis of some chronic diseases, including CKD, which leads to deterioration of the condition of patients, complications of the disease, disability and, unfortunately, death of patients [77; p. 22-26]

The development of the system of nephrological care and renal replacement therapy (RRT) is not able to solve the problem of treating patients and improving their quality of life. There is a need for a universal, simple and convenient methodological framework that allows you to combine the efforts of many clinicians-nephrologists, cardiologists, endocrinologists, therapists and others for the purpose of early diagnosis of chronic kidney pathology of different nature, timely appointment of nephroprotective therapy and nephroprophylaxis. [70; pp. 22-26;]

The initial attempt to address these issues was initiated at the beginning of the XXI century by the National Kidney Foundation of the United States (NationalKidneyFoundation-NKF). The analysis of the results of numerous studies on the diagnosis and treatment of kidney diseases, the prognostic role of a number of indicators, and terminological concepts formed the basis of the concept of CKD (Chron-ickidneydisease – CKD) [54; p. 4-26]. Later, experts from the European Kidney Association, the European Association for Dialysis and Transplantation (ERA-EDTA), and KDIGO (KidneyDisease:ImprovingGlobalOutcomes) participated in the development of this model [38; p 950-957].

Currently, the concept of CKD and its proposed classification have received worldwide recognition by scientists and specialists in the field of nephrology.

In 2002, the National Kidney Foundation of the United States published practical recommendations for the identification and management of patients with CKD - K/DOQIGuideline (KidneyDiseaseOutcomesQualityInitiative). These recommendations address the assessment, classification and stratification of CKD risk [62; p 107-114]

Recommendations include the study of the degree of renal damage by determining the albumin / creatinine ratio, evaluating the glomerular filtration rate (GFR) by blood creatinine level using calculated formulas. Since the prevalence of early stages of CKD in the general population is quite high, the recommendations created are useful not only for nephrologists, but also for doctors of other specialties – cardiologists, endocrinologists and general practitioners [34; 48].

In 2008, in the UK, the National Institute for Health and Clinical Excellence (NICE - NationalInstituteforClinicalExcellence) established guidelines for the early diagnosis and management of CKD in adults in primary and secondary care [27; 53]

In 2012, Australia created its own CARI (CaringforAustralianswithRenalImpairment) recommendations [58; p 1-32].

CKD is a growing public health problem in all countries of the world due to the huge increase in its risk factors in recent years. Due to rapid lifestyle changes, there is a significant increase in the prevalence of risk factors that are the main causes of CKD.

Epidemiological assessment followed by prioritization of risk factors helps to determine the prevalence and incidence of CKD, and these studies are necessary for the development of prevention programs.

To this end, screening studies are being implemented worldwide to determine the local burden of chronic kidney disease and its contribution to public health.

According to studies conducted in different countries of the world, the following figures are determined: according to the results of the NHANES study conducted in 2005-2010, signs of CKD are observed in 14-20% of the US population, according to the KEEP epidemiological study conducted in 2000-2011, the incidence of CKD among the adult population of the United States is 23.8%. According to the results of the national epidemiological study "Beijingstudy", conducted in China in 2008, CKD is observed in 14% of the country's residents. In 2013, such a national epidemiological study was implemented in India (SEEK – India, 2013). According to this survey, CKD occurs in 17.2% of Indian residents. The prevalence of CKD among residents of the Congo was 12.4%, with the most unfavorable stages of the disease observed in 8% of residents (in the United States -15.7%).

In Russia, a huge epidemiological study on the definition of CKD has not been conducted, but scientific studies conducted in certain categories of the population confirm that in older age groups CKD was observed in 66.3%, among patients suffering from pathologies of the cardiovascular system, the incidence of CKD was 16%.

The first epidemiological study of kidney disease in Kazakhstan was conducted in 1980 and studied the incidence of nosological types of kidney diseases. The results of the screening survey conducted among students of Karaganda universities showed that 13.6 % of students have pathological changes in urine characteristic of the early stages of CKD. [36; p. 6-16].

According to the scientific literature, it is determined that large-scale epidemiological studies for the realization of the prevalence of CKD among the population of our Republic have not been conducted. However, a study was conducted in separate groups of patients with certain pathologies aimed at studying the clinical and genetic features of nephropathy in diabetes mellitus and metabolic syndrome and the development of CKD in patients with arterial hypertension.

According to Kamilov D. N. (2011), the average level of disability due to nephrological diseases in Tashkent is 0.5 per 10,000 population, the main part was made up of women of reproductive age (84.5%) and the working-age population (70.5%).

Scientific surveys of Daminova K. M. and Kayumov U. K. (2011) show that type 2 diabetes is a risk factor for the development of CKD. Analysis of the results of a scientific study showed a high incidence of nephropathy in direct-line relatives of patients suffering from type 2 diabetes mellitus complicated by diabetic nephropathy.

In families of patients with metabolic syndrome, nephropathy occurs in every third (35.5%).

Studies have shown that CKD is a serious medical and social problem that significantly affects the health of people and the economic condition of the country on all continents [28; 51]. The most obvious consequence of CKD is the high cost of life-saving RRT (dialysis and kidney transplantation), which places a heavy burden on the health system.

In the United States, 28.9% of Medicare's budget was spent on non-RRT CKD patients, who accounted for 12.7% of the total number of people covered by Medicare, in 2011. The need for hospitalization in patients with CKD is 38% higher compared to people without CKD, and mortality is 43% higher[39; pp. 39-44].

The high prevalence, adverse outcomes, and complications of CKD give reason to raise the issue of the feasibility of developing and implementing measures for its early detection, nephroprotection, and nephroprophylaxis [70; pp. 1-70].

CKD occupies a special place in the family of chronic non-communicable diseases (CKD). Most cases of CKD are secondary kidney lesions within other CKD diseases, such as diabetes mellitus and hypertension. This is one of the reasons that most of the risk factors for CKD are shared with the risk factors for these diseases, so programs for the prevention and early detection of diabetes mellitus and arterial hypertension play a crucial role in the prevention of CKD [60; p.71-87].

The results of the NHANESIII study [24; p. 601 - 609] demonstrated that in addition to arterial hypertension and diabetes mellitus, the main factors for the development of CKD are also the age of patients. Studies have found that, in 11% of people over 65 years of age without arterial hypertension and diabetes mellitus, CKD of stages III-V of development is determined [36; p. 6-16].

The characteristic general aging of the population in developed countries significantly affects the increase in the prevalence of CKD, which in most cases is associated with an increase in the number of patients with vascular kidney damage [15; p.17-20].

Recent publications prove that a large number of patients with arterial hypertension, hyperlipidemia and diabetes mellitus have a high risk of developing kidney failure. This fact is proved by the research of Tangri, N. etal. [56; p. 514-520], which indicates that about 40% of the adult population has an increased risk of developing CKD and renal dysfunction.

The formation of a healthy lifestyle of the population reduces the risk of developing CKD, as well as other CKD. However, it is important to emphasize that the common risk factors for CKD - high blood pressure, dyslipidemia, smoking, poor nutrition, inactivity, reduced carbohydrate tolerance, obesity, alcohol consumption increases the risk of not only secondary nephropathies, but CKD in general. A decrease in the effect of these risk factors leads to a decrease in these pathologies and their complications. [65; pp. 7-17].

Playing a central role in the regulation of metabolism and the elimination of its end products from the body, exotoxins of the kidneys functionally and structurally suffer from an irrational diet and an unhealthy lifestyle of the population [68; p 117-124].

It should be emphasized that non - compliance with the diet, heavy consumption of fatty, salty and spicy foods directly correlates with the development of kidney pathology, especially in adults. In this regard, many authors agree that poor nutrition is also an important risk factor for the formation and development of CKD.

According to these national guidelines, risk factors for the progression of CKD include a number of chronic diseases, such as diabetes mellitus, arterial hypertension, autoimmune diseases, various pathogenic and opportunistic microbes, urinary tract stones, lower urinary tract obstruction, kidney surgery, frequent use of analgesics and other nephrotoxic drugs, acute renal failure, a history of nephropathy in pregnant women, obesity, hyperhomocysteinemia, a violation of calcium-phosphorus metabolism, which are divided into modifiable and non-modifiable.

1.2. Risk factors for CKD-a medical and social problem.

It is known that CKD is a supranosological concept that unites all patients with signs of kidney damage that persist for 3 or more months according to laboratory and instrumental studies and / or a decrease in function estimated by the value of GFR [66; pp. 89-115].

For the diagnosis of CKD, in addition to clinical and instrumental studies, it is necessary to determine the markers of renal damage and the state of renal function. The most accessible, simple and cheap laboratory method for the study of markers of renal damage is a general urinalysis, which allows detecting proteinuria, hematuria, leukocyturia and other indicators of the pathological process in a single portion of urine [46; pp. 89-115, 62; c17-28]. Along with the advantage of this method, there are certain disadvantages associated with the imperfections of this method. The imperfections of this method include insufficient accuracy, especially when the level of proteinuria is below 0.5 g/l. A normal result of the general analysis of the patient's urine does not exclude the presence of CKD [52; p.38-43]. All the diagnostic criteria developed to date for determining kidney pathology are aimed at determining two components of signs – kidney damage and a decrease in GFR.

It is important to emphasize that at the beginning of the development of CKD, kidney function can remain intact for a long time, despite the presence of pronounced signs of damage. In normal or elevated GFR, as well as in patients with its initial decrease (60 < GFR<90 ml / min/1.73 m2), the presence of signs of kidney damage is a prerequisite for the diagnosis of CKD[35; pp. 727-733].

The detection of GFR in patients with more than 120 ml / min/1.73 m2 is also considered a deviation from the normal parameters for the kidneys, since in individuals suffering from diabetes mellitus and obesity, it may reflect the phenomenon of hyperfiltration caused by their increased perfusion with the development of glomerular hypertension, which leads to their functional overload, damage with further sclerosis of the structure [44; pp. 16-27].

However, to date, increased glomerular filtration (GFR > 120 ml / min/1.73 m2) is not included by specialists among the independent diagnostic criteria for CKD, but is considered a risk factor for its development [47; p.5-8].

The presence of CKD in diabetes mellitus and obesity is indicated by markers of renal damage, primarily increased albuminuria in patients[52; pp. 38-43].

There are 5 stages of CKD, depending on the level of GFR. Patients with stage III CKD are the most common among the population, while this group is heterogeneous in terms of the risk of cardiovascular complications, which increases with a decrease in GFR. Therefore, stage III of CKD was proposed to be divided into two sub - stages-IIIA and IIIB. [47; pp. 5-8].

If we talk about the classification of CKD, we want to highlight the fact that there were numerous classifications of various pathological conditions of the kidneys. These classifications emphasized the nature of the pathology, the form of the disease, the duration of the pathological process, and so on, but they did not give a complete picture of the course and outcome of the disease.

Currently, clinicians use a single classification of CKD, given in the International Classification of Diseases 10-revision (ICD-10) 2007.

CKD in ICD-10 (2007) is presented as follows:

18.1 CKD - C1 stage, GFR level>90 ml / min/1.73 m2

18.2 CKD - C2 stage, GFR level 60-89 ml / min/1.73 m2

18.3 CKD - C3a stage, GFR level 45-59 ml / min/1.73 m2

18.3 CKD - C3b stage, GFR level 30-44 ml / min/1.73 m2

18.4 CKD - C4 stage, GFR level 15-29 ml / min/1.73 m2

18.5 CKD - C5 stage, GFR level<15 ml / min/1.73 m2

18.9 Unspecified CKD

If we talk about the strategy for identifying chronic kidney disease, a deep analysis of modern domestic and foreign literature sources, as well as clinical practice, shows that there is no consensus among specialists on this issue. There are numerous recommendations that are not perfect.

But a large number of researchers are inclined to believe that screening studies are the most optimal and recommend this method to be more acceptable for the detection of CKD. In this regard, various strategies have been proposed to identify it [23; 32, 62].

However, not all researchers share a common view and screening programs in their CKD studies are accepted not everywhere The published evidence base for CKD compared to that for cardiovascular disease and diabetes mellitus is limited, and to date there are not enough randomized controlled trials to compare the effectiveness of CKD screening with its effectiveness.

The goal of screening programs has almost always been to identify CKD at an early stage of the pathological process, which will allow for a timely final diagnosis and start appropriate nephroprotective treatment.

A great help in assessing the need for laboratory tests is provided by special questionnaires that the subjects fill out independently or with the help of secondary medical personnel. The most well-known questionnaire created in the United States for the KEEP study [162; p. 107-114], dedicated to the screening and monitoring of individuals with CKD risk factors. Based on the data of the American epidemiological study NHANES in the USA, an improved questionnaire SCORED (SCreeningforOccultREnalDisease) was developed [33; 38].

It should be noted that currently in many countries of the world there are so - called screening centers for CKD, created with the support of the state or charitable foundations, in which everyone who wants to be examined can pass a free questionnaire and interview for the presence of risk factors for CKD, in addition, they can pass the necessary laboratory tests.

With the introduction of modern means of informatization of IT technologies in medicine, this way of detecting CKD becomes more accessible. The prospects of using IT technologies for screening studies are shown by the results of the analysis of 1032 case histories in one of the central district hospitals of the Moscow region of the Russian Federation, which showed that among working-age patients undergoing examination and treatment in therapeutic departments and without a diagnosis of kidney disease, GFR < 60 ml/min/1.73 m2, that is, CKD 3a-5, was observed in 16% of cases. And in a sample of patients with cardiovascular diseases

A prerequisite after the completion of screening studies, according to many experts, is not only the identification of the patient with CKD, but also the inclusion of him in the risk group. In the future, these patients should undergo a mandatory primary consultation with a nephrologist in order to make a nosological diagnosis, select etiotropic, pathogenetic and nephroprotective therapy, as well as carry out secondary preventive measures for the progression of this pathology.

1.3 Diagnostic criteria and current strategies for the detection of chronic kidney disease

Practice shows that laboratory indicators or markers of kidney damage in patients most often include proteinuria, changes in urine sediment, blood and urine tests, changes in functional and imaging methods of research, characteristic of violations of certain partial kidney functions [54; p .4-26].

At the same time, it is known that the early (preclinical) stages of chronic kidney dysfunction, corresponding mainly to stages 1-2, and sometimes to stages 3 of CKD, are characterized by an asymptomatic or low-symptom course in the current NKF classification [136; p.33-40]. Obvious clinical changes, including detected proteinuria, as well as structural changes in the organ during its ultrasound imaging, as a rule, indicate a far-reaching, irreversible pathological process [24].

According to the overwhelming majority of authors, in clinical practice, in the absence of any other signs of chronic kidney damage, the level of albuminuria is the only and relatively early indicator that allows us to exclude or confirm the presence of a subclinical course of CKD, especially in conditions of preserved GFR [52; pp. 38-43].

Studies have shown that albuminuria / proteinuria in the concept of CKD-K / DOQI is considered as a marker of renal dysfunction [16; p. 89-115, 17; c19-21].

At the KDIGO London Conference in 2009, the previous gradations of the severity of albuminuria ("stages of albuminuria") were left:
- less than 30 mg of albumin in the urine
- 30-299 mg of albumin in the urine
- 300 mg or more of albumin in the urine [56; pp. 89-115].

To assess albuminuria/proteinuria as part of a screening study, an albuminuria test or a general urinalysis can be used from laboratory parameters, which includes determining the concentration of total protein in the urine. The albuminuria test has an advantage for the early detection of CKD, since it is more sensitive and allows us to differentiate all 3 categories of albuminuria in the examined patients [30; pp. 33-38].

The albuminuria test is of particular value in the early diagnosis of CKD in the examined patients with hypertension, diabetes mellitus and obesity, in which the appearance of significant proteinuria is observed only at the late stages of the pathological process [30; p.33-38, 65; p. 7-17].

The analysis of the literature showed that albuminuria is detected in 20-30% of people with arterial hypertension, in 25-40% of patients with type I or II diabetes, in 5-7% of people in the general population of the conditionally healthy population [59; pp. 1517-1523]. The development of albuminuria is associated with almost all components of the metabolic syndrome and is also noted in tobacco smoking [11].

The most rational and reliable way to determine GFR in routine laboratory practice is to automatically calculate it in biochemical laboratories, which should produce 2 results – serum creatinine concentration and calculated GFR [11].

The formulas proposed for practical health care take into account the peculiarities of creatinine kinetics due to age, different muscle mass and increased tubular creatinine secretion in the late stages of CKD. When the creatinine level falls within the reference (normal) laboratory values, GFR can be reduced to a level corresponding to the 3a and even 3b stages of CKD [63];

To date , the CKD-EPI method of GFR calculation is used for screening, taking into account the level of creatinine in the blood serum, gender and age of the patient. There are nomograms for determining GFR by this method. Electronic calculators are available for calculating GFR on-line or using separate applications for personal computers and mobile devices. Currently, the use of the old Cockcroft - Gault equations is not recommended for calculating GFR in practical medicine [64; 1-70].

Thus, our in-depth analysis of the literature sources of domestic and foreign authors has shown that the prevalence of CKD in the world is quite high, which leads to a deterioration in the quality of life of patients and high mortality among patients.

For the early detection of CKD, the authors proposed screening studies and successfully carried out these works. Optimal classification introduction optimal methods of clinical examination and laboratory diagnostics are given. In addition, a strategy for the detection of CKD is proposed and risk factors for the progression of this pathology are described. Attention is drawn to the work devoted to the determination and evaluation of albuminuria glomerular filtration rate in the diagnosis of CKD. It is proved that a successful solution to the problem of CKD only by RRT is impossible.

At the same time, the problems of early diagnosis of CKD with the help of screening studies in rural areas, the determination of risk factors for the development and progression of CKD in this category of individuals, modern methods of early diagnosis and prediction of the course of CKD with the help of ST-technologies have not yet been solved, an algorithm for preventing the formation and development of CKD in the adult population has not been developed.

In connection with the above, the continuation of research work in this area is relevant and in demand.

CHAPTER II. SCOPE AND DESIGN OF RESEARCH, MATERIALS AND METHODS

To study the assessment of diagnostic predictors of the formation and development of chronic kidney disease, it is necessary to conduct not only clinical, but also laboratory and socio-medical studies. In this regard, the research will have to be carried out in several stages. Given this, we have described the design of the study and selected a sufficient amount of research.

§ 2.1. Research design

The implementation of this research work was carried out in 3 stages:

Stage 1. Selection of the research object, determination of the research volume and population, distribution into representative groups, organization of randomized trials.

Stage 2. Conducting screening studies in selected localities of urban areas with the help of a specially developed "Questionnaire for identifying the risk of developing chronic kidney disease".

Stage 3. In-depth clinical, instrumental and laboratory studies of patients in whom diagnostic predictors (criteria) were identified during screening studies) CKD. Statistical processing, comparative analysis of the material and development of ways to prevent the progression of CKD.

§ 2.2. Research materials

At the first stage, the object, the contingent, and the scope of research were selected. To achieve this goal, the studies were conducted in the city family polyclinics No. 3, No. 5 and No. 11 of the city of Bukhara

87 women of childbearing age were involved in the research work. The medical examination of the population and the survey-interview of this contingent were carried out in an outpatient setting located on this territory.

At the second stage of the study, screening studies were conducted. The medical examination of the population was accompanied by a survey-interview and the completion of a specially developed goal "Questionnaire for identifying the risk of developing chronic kidney disease" and the determination of microalbumin in a single portion of urine by a semi-quantitative method using test strips.

The questionnaire consists of 2 parts: the passport part and the main part. The passport part consists of 6 questions that include materials about this person. The main part consists of 40 questions that are designed to identify risk factors for the formation and development of CKD. Questions related to age, gender, place of work, the presence of concomitant diseases and conditions, adherence to a healthy lifestyle, anthropometric data, and other aspects.

The occurrence of various pathologies of other organs leading to the formation and development of CKD as risk factors for the development of this pathology is analyzed.

At the third stage of the study in this selected contingent(n=87), which included: identification of anamnesis of life and illness; determination of height and weight indicators-height (cm), weight (kg), waist circumference (OT), hip circumference (OB), waist-to – hip ratio (OT/OB), waist-to-height ratio (OT/height), body mass index (BMI) according to the Kettle formula (depending on why the normal body weight was allocated BMI18,5-24,9 kg/m2, excess weight). weight-BMI 25-29. 9 kg/m2 and obese BMI ≥ 30 kg/m2.

The basis for the diagnosis of CKD, as a consequence of structural or functional disorders, is cases of deviation in the laboratory and functional results of the study, which were preserved for more than 3 months after the initial detection of the disease by the method of the most detailed examination.

Microalbuminuria (MAU> 10 mg/L) was detected in 61 of these patients in this group. In 23 (37.7±4.52%), the glomerular filtration rate (GFR) < 90 ml / min was 1.73 m2, which allowed us to state the I-III stages of CKD (K/DOOL, 2002).

The design of this study is presented in Table 2.1.

Table 2.1.

Stages and scope of research in the surveyed population permanently residing in urban areas (n=87)

Stages	I	II	III
Informed consent of the patient to the study	+	+	+
Anamnesis of life and illness		+	+
Physical examination		+	+
Filling out the questionnaire		+	
Determination of BMI		+	
Clinical and biochemical blood tests		+	+
General urinalysis		+	+
Determination of microalbumin and creatinine in urine		+	+
Clinical blood test			

Biochemical blood analysis (ALT, AST, total protein, lipid fraction, glucose)			+
Determination of urea, serum creatinine and GFR			+
Determination of coagulogram parameters			+
Ultrasound of the genitourinary system and pelvis			+

Patients who have identified diagnostic criteria for CKD (microalbuminuria, low GFR) were examined for 2-3 months after a comprehensive examination to clarify the diagnosis of CKD in a specialized clinic in the city of Bukhara.

When performing the research, we followed all the ethical principles of human-assisted medical research adopted by the Helsinki Declaration of the World Medical Association in 1964 (the latest addition at the 59th General Assembly of the World Medical Association in 2008 in Seoul).

The research was carried out on the basis of the Department of Faculty and Hospital Therapy of the Bukhara State Medical Institute in the period from 2011 to 2017.

§ 2.3. Research methods

General clinical examination: Traditional clinical examinations were conducted to examine therapeutic patients. Anthropometric indicators were evaluated: height, weight, OT, OB, BMI according to the Kettle formula: BMI (kg/m2)= weight (kg)/height (m2) (Table 2.2).

Table 2.1.

Classification of obesity by BMI (WHO, 1997)

Types of body weight	BMI, kg / m2	Risk of comorbidities
Body weight deficit	<18,5	Low (increased risk)

Normal body weight	18,5-24,9	Usual
Overweight	25,0-29,9	Elevated
Grade I obesity	30,0-34,9	Tall
Grade II obesity	35,0-39,9	Very high
Grade III obesity	>40	Extremely high

- Measurement blood pressure (BP) was measured in the morning, in the patient's sitting position at least 3 times, with the calculation of the average value of systolic blood pressure and diastolic blood pressure. The criteria for arterial hypertension were systolic blood pressure ≥ 140 mmHg and diastolic blood pressure ≥ 90 mmHg, or normal blood pressure levels against the background of constant antihypertensive medication. The severity of arterial hypertension was determined according to the classification of hypertension according to the recommendations of the IOC:
- 1 degree of AH – 130-159 and / or 80-100 mm Hg
- 2 degree-160-180 and / or 100-109 mm Hg
- 3 degree -180 and/or 100 mm Hg and above.

Ultrasound examination: All the examined patients underwent ultrasound examination of the kidneys using special equipment of the company "ToshibaSSA-340" (Japan) with a sensor frequency of 3.5 MHz.

The purpose of ultrasound is to determine the location of the kidneys and their mobility, shape, contours, linear and volumetric parameters; to determine the clarity of the image, the thickness of the fibrous capsule and adipose tissue; the state of the parenchyma - the thickness, density, clarity of differentiation of the cortical, medullary layers, parenchyma and renal sinus; the state of the cavity system - expansion or deformation, the degree of dilation, the thickness of the walls of the upper, middle and lower groups of cups; to determine the paranephral fiber, own vessels and main retroperitoneal, adjacent organs - the adrenal glands, ureter and bladder.

Determination of the main parameters of hemostasis

The device "HumanClotJunior" coagulometer, manufactured in 2013, by "HumanGesellschaftBiochemicaundDiagnostica" (Wiesbaden, Germany) was used. Conducting a study of clotting with the structure of fibrin, using the endpoint method. The following tests were performed: PV (Prothrombin Time) - expressed in seconds, can be converted to % and the calculated method is determined by INR; APTT (Activated Partial Thromboplastin Time) - expressed in seconds; Fibrinogen- expressed in seconds, automatically converted to mg/dl concentration in peripheral blood plasma.

Determination of hematological parameters

To determine the parameters of peripheral blood, an automatic hematological analyzer BC-5800 from MindrayCo.Ltd (China) was used, which is able to determine 29 parameters + 2 histograms +2 scategrams, differentiation of white blood cells by 5 parameters.

Determination of biochemical parameters

For this purpose, an automatic biochemical analyzer VS - 200 from MINDRAY (China) was used.

Creatinine was determined using a photocolorimetric test for kinetic measurement, without deproteinization. The principle of the method: creatinine in an alkaline solution of orange-red color in a complex with picric acid. The absorption of this complex is proportional to the creatinine concentration in the sample (Test "HumanGesellschaftBiochemicaundDiagnostica", Wiesbaden, Germany).

Urea was determined using the enzyme colorimetric method. The test "HumanGesellschaftBiochemicaundDiagnostica" (Wiesbaden, Germany) was used.

Albumin was determined by using bromocresol green. Bromocresol green forms a colored complex with albumin in the citrate buffer. The absorption of the resulting complex is proportional to the albumin concentration in the sample. (Test «HumanGesellschaftBiochemicaundDiagnostica»,Wiesbaden, Germany).

Glucose was determined after its conversion under the action of hexokinase to gluconate-6-phosphate and subsequent interaction of glucose-6-phosphate with NAD in the presence of glucose-6-phosphate dehydrogenase. The increase in the optical density of the solution is proportional to the concentration of glucose in the sample. (Test «HumanGesellschaftBiochemicaundDiagnostica»,Wiesbaden, Germany).

Cholesterol was determined after enzymatic hydrolysis and oxidation. The H_2O_2 formed as a result of these reactions reacts under the action of peroxidase with 4-aminophenazone and phenol to form a colored product-quinonimine (Test "HumanGesellschaftBiochemicaundDiagnostica", Wiesbaden, Germany).

The concentration of triglycerides was determined after enzymatic hydrolysis under the action of lipase. Formed as a result of a series of enzymatic reactions, H_2O_2 reacts with 4-aminoantipyrine and 4-chlorophenol under the action of peroxidase to form a colored quinonimine(Test "HumanGesellschaftBiochemicaundDiagnostica",Wiesbaden, Germany).

Low - density lipoprotein (LDL) - the quantitative determination of LDL cholesterol consists of two stages: the first stage is the removal of the chylomicrons of VLDL cholesterol and HDL cholesterol from the reaction zone under the action of enzymes.

Determination of urine parameters

A general urine analysis was performed using Combina 13 test strips on a Combineyzer urinary analyzer (Germany).

Test strips for determining the biochemical parameters of urine, 13-parameter. The principle of the test: reflective photometry (visual evaluation) of the result on a color scale. Test parameters: blood (hemoglobin), bilirubin, urobilinogen, ketones, protein, nitrites, glucose, pH, specific gravity, white blood cells, ascorbic acid, microalbumin, creatinine, albumin/creatinine ratio . Lower limit of determination: blood – 10 red blood cells/mcl, bilirubin – 1 mg/dl, urobilinogen – 0.2 mg/dl, ketones – 5 mg/dl, protein – 30 mg/dl, glucose – 50 mg/dl, white blood cells - 15 white blood cells/mcl, ascorbic acid – 10 mg/dl, microalbumin – 10 mg/dl, creatinine – 10 mg/dl Test strips are used for rapid determination (determination time 1 minute) in the urine, bilirubin, urobilinogen, ketones, glucose, protein, blood (red blood cells/hemoglobin), pH, nitrites, white blood cells, specific gravity/density, ascorbic acid, creatinine, microalbumin.

Determination of the concentration of albumin in the urine was carried out using test strips Combina 13 manufactured by "Humang GmbH" (Germany) and Urine-2AC manufactured by "CypressDiagnostics" (Belgium). Diagnostic strips are designed for semi-quantitative measurement of the concentration of albumin in the urine using the analyzer "Combineyzer 13". The test for measuring albumin in urine is based on the binding of a dye using sulfonephthalene. The resulting color ranges from pale green to the color of a blue moon.

The level of albuminuria was assessed on the following scale: 10 mg/l-optimal or slight increase, 10-29 mg/l – moderate increase, 30-80 mg/l – high, > 150 mg /l – very high.

In order to clarify the diagnostic reliability of test strips for urine analysis in 20 patients at the same time, proteinuria was determined using two methods: the determination of microalbumin in daily urine and the determination of microalbumin in a single morning portion of urine. The difference between the indicators of these methods was as follows: MAU in daily urine averaged 69.16 mg / day. MAU in a single urine morning portion averaged 64.66 mg/day.

Determination of creatinine concentration in the urine. This test is based on the reaction of creatinine with a dye-metal complex. In an alkaline environment, creatinine reacts with the dye-metal complex to form a purple-brown complex.

Statistical methods

Statistical analysis of the obtained results was carried out using the methods of variation statistics. The reliability of the differences in the mean values was estimated on the basis of the Student's test (t) with the calculation of the probability of error (P) when checking the normality of the distribution and the equality of the general variances (F – Fisher's test). The correlation analysis was performed using Spearman (Rs) and Pearson (r) methods.

In conclusion, I would like to emphasize that for this purpose, the object and the research contingent were correctly selected in compliance with all the rules of the general and sample population.

Almost all selected respondents and survey groups were representative, and all studies were randomized.

Statistical methods are also carried out in accordance with the high requirements of statistical analysis.

All of the above allows you to indicate that the results obtained are reliable, and the conclusions are true.

CHAPTER III ANALYSIS OF THE RESULTS OF THE STUDY BY FREQUENCY PREVALENCE OF CHRONIC KIDNEY DISEASE IN WOMEN OF FERTIL AGE

About 10% of the world's adult population suffers from CKD, including nearly 200 million women worldwide. The diagnosis is made in the presence of any chronic kidney damage, even if their function is not impaired. The progression of CKD does not always occur, but in many cases, deterioration of kidney function is observed for several years or even months and leads to the need for dialysis [56; p. 52-56].

Screening is a secondary prevention measure aimed at identifying a specific disease in the preclinical stage. During screening, a mass examination of a contingent from certain risk groups is carried out, who do not consider themselves sick, do not seek medical help and, accordingly, do not receive specific treatment. The main purpose of screening is to detect the disease before specific clinical symptoms appear and to completely cure the pathology [46; p. 52-56, 124; p.601-609].

It should be emphasized that the results of screening studies in rural areas of our republic are rare. In this regard, we considered it appropriate to conduct a survey of the population living permanently in rural areas for the early detection of CKD.

The methods of screening examination and the place of residence of patients were described in detail in chapter II, so we did not consider it appropriate to dwell on this.

The main selection criterion was microalbuminuria (MAU >10 mg / L), which persisted for 3 months or more, considering this parameter a diagnostic predictor of CKD development. Among the examined patients, this criterion of CKD was detected in 27 persons (31±4.9%) out of 87 examined patients.

On the basis of clinical materials, parameters of laboratory and instrumental studies, the diagnosis was established in some subjects, the number of examined and identified nosological units differed from each other, as in 1 examined patient, sometimes there were 2 or 3 established diagnoses of the disease. Thus, in 87 patients with diagnoses established on the basis of outpatient records, there were 101 diseases (1.15 nosologies per 1 examined person). The contingent with the diagnosis established after our examination (n=27) had 50 nosologies – 1.86 per 1 examined person.accordingly, the data in Table 3.1. are calculated from the total number of identified nosological units.

Table 3.1

Indicators of the frequency of occurrence of various pathologies that were risk factors for the development of chronic kidney disease,%

Nosological units	DIAGNOSIS	
	established on the basis of outpatient charts of 101 nosology n=87	installed after the survey 50 nosology n=27
Arterial hypertension	37/42,5±4,93	9/33,33±4,72* ↓
Coronary heart disease	13/15,4±3,60	4/14,81±2,53 ↔
Diabetes mellitus	5/5,74±2,83	2/7,4±2,13* ↓
Rheumatological diseases	7/7,71±2,66	2/7,4±2,13 ↔
Anemia of various degrees	11/12,64±2,57	1/3,7±1,86* ↔
Endemic goiter	3/3,51±1,66	4/14,81±2,53 ↔
Obesity	11/12,5±1,18	5/18,55±3,88* ↑

Note: in the numerator absolute, in the denominator relative (%) indicators: * - a sign of a significant difference in the parameter; ↑ ↓ and ↔ - an increase, decrease or absence of a difference in the indicator from the compared group

Among the established diagnoses, both on the basis of outpatient records and after examination, diseases of the cardiovascular system were often encountered, with arterial hypertension, respectively, 42.5±4.93%, (n=37) and 33.33±4.72%, (n=9), coronary heart disease, respectively, 15.4±3.60%, (n=13) and 14.81±2.53%, (n=4)

Other established diagnoses were less frequent - diabetes mellitus, respectively, 5.74±2.83%, (n=5) and 7.4±2.13%, (n=2), rheumatic diseases, respectively, 7.71±2.66%, (n=27) and 7.4±2.13 % (n=2), anemia, respectively, 12.64±2.57%, (n=11) and 3.7±1.86%, (n=1), endemic goiter, respectively, 3.51±1.66%, (n=3) and 14.81±2.53%, (n=4), obese, respectively, 12.5±1.18%, (n=11) and 18.55±3.888%, (n=5).

We can say that among the above-mentioned diseases, the level of diagnosis of obesity as a nosological unit is very low - the difference between the groups is 6.2 times. This indicates that health professionals do not assess obesity as an unfavorable risk factor for the development of various pathological conditions, including CKD.

Given the importance of urinary tract diseases as risk factors for CKD, we decided to give the frequency of these nosological units separately (Table 3.2)

Table 3.2.

Indicators frequency of occurrence of urinary tract diseases as risk factors for CKD in the examined population

Nosological units	Диагноз	
	established on the basis of outpatient card data, n=21	established after the survey, n=40
Pyelonephritis	10/47,06±4,99	22/55,17±4,97*↑
Cystitis (acute and chronic)	7/35,29±4,77	9/24,14±4,27* ↓
Urolithiasis	3/13,73±3,44	9/20,69±4,05 ↔
Glomerulonephritis	1/3,92±1,94	0

Note: in the numerator absolute, in the denominator relative (%) indicators: * - a sign of a significant difference in the parameter; ↑ ↓ and ↔ - an increase, decrease or absence of a difference in the indicator from the compared group

It should be noted that among the examined patients, who were diagnosed on the basis of outpatient records, the diagnosis of CKD as a nosological unit was not detected. After the examination, this diagnosis was established in 29.1% (n=21) of the respondents from the general subjects.

In our studies, each separately, the role of these nosological units listed in Table 3.2. as a risk factor for CKD is insignificant, so we decided to use the general group of urinary tract diseases to determine the groups at risk for CKD.

The conducted scientific studies prove that hypertension, diabetes mellitus, and obesity are traditional factors of CKD development [4; pp. 82-87]. But in the development of chronic kidney damage, non-traditional factors of CKD development are of great importance. The results of our research show that these factors include the place of residence, ethnic customs of the people, the way and standard of living of the population, the effectiveness of preventive measures carried out by medical institutions of widespread non - communicable chronic diseases, the use of poor-quality drinking water, violation of the rules of rational nutrition, constant consumption of high-calorie food by the population.

According to ValerieA and KathrinR [2017], which conducted studies in Switzerland, many of the factors we mentioned were the main causes of the spread of CKD in the population.

Thus, it was found that there is a significant difference between the established diagnoses based on the outpatient records of rural family clinics and after our examination. Arterial hypertension, diabetes mellitus, obesity and urinary tract diseases, which were among the main risk factors for the development of CKD, were not sufficiently identified in the primary and repeated treatment of patients for medical care.

Based on this , to determine the frequency of non-traditional risk factors that affect the development and progression of CKD, the following factors were analyzed using the integration method:

- abuse of nephrotoxic drugs that are usually sold without a prescription in our country - analgesics, nonsteroidal anti-inflammatory drugs (NSAIDs), some

antibiotics;
- abuse of salty and bitter foods;
- bad habits - smoking, drinking alcohol;
- non-controlling pathological conditions and diseases with a history of history (proteinuria, dysuria, nephropathy of pregnant women, arterial hypertension of pregnant women, acute allergic reactions, acute bleeding with hypovolemia);
- chronic foci of infection - chronic tonsillitis, chronic otitis media, dental caries;

When analyzing the frequency of occurrence of these factors, we paid attention to the level of identification and / or elimination of these factors as the cause of the development of other diseases (Table 3.3)

Table 3.3

The frequency of occurrence of non-traditional factors as a risk factor for CKD among the examined patients

Non-traditional factors		Diagnosis	
		established on the basis of outpatient card data, n=21	established after the survey, n=40
Abuse of nephrotoxic drugs		13/58,57±4,92	25/62,61±4,83 ↔
Abuse of salty and bitter foods		7/33,80±4,73	17/42,99±4,95 ↔
A history of proteinuria		4/20,95±4,16	15/38,31±4,86*↑
Nephropathy of pregnant women^		12/60,90±4,87	24/60,0±4,89 ↔
Arterial hypertension in pregnancy^		8/39,09±4,87	16/40,0±4,89 ↔
The presence of chronic	Chronic tonsillitis	6/31,90±4,66	15/38,31±4,86 ↔
	Chronic otitis media	1/1,90±1,36	1/5,60±2,29 ↔

| foci of infection | Dental caries | 12/58,57±4,92 | 25/64,48±4,78 ↔ |

Note: ^-indicators are calculated based on the number of women examined in the groups n=21 and n=60, respectively; * - a sign of a significant difference in the parameter; ↑ ↓ and ↔ - an increase, decrease or absence of a difference in the indicator from the compared group

Among non-traditional risk factors for CKD are often met abuse of nephrotoxic drugs (analgesics, NSAIDs, antibiotics), respectively 58,57±4,92% (n=13) and 62,61±4,83% (n=25); the presence of chronic foci of infection, of which a large number of identified caries 58,57±4,92% (n=12) and 64,48±4,78% (n=25), and in the next place chronic tonsillitis work at 31.90±4,66% (n=6) and 38,31±4,86% (n=15); among surveyed women residing in the rural municipality of residence of non-traditional factors in the development of CKD identified nephropathy pregnant women in history, respectively 60,90±4,87%(n=12) and 60,0±4,89% (n=24).

Analysis of the results shows that the above factors are not fully evaluated as a risk factor for CKD and the effectiveness of preventive measures for non-communicable chronic diseases among the rural population is quite low.

Thus, the frequency of non-traditional CKD risk factors among the subjects varies, ranging from 1.90±1.36% (chronic otitis media) to 58.57±4.92% (abuse of nephrotic drugs). Of the 10 non-traditional risk factors studied, the most significant in the group of patients diagnosed on the basis of outpatient records were abuse of nephrotoxic drugs (58.57%), dysuria of unclear etiology (43.80%), abuse of salty and bitter foods (33.40%), bad habits (21.42%), proteinuria in the anamnesis (20.95%) and nephropathy of pregnant women in the anamnesis (60.90%). Almost the same trend in the occurrence of non-traditional risk factors was observed in the group with established diagnoses during screening tests. From the findings, it follows that, first, the population permanently living in rural areas generally have the same non-traditional risk factors for CKD; second, the population is not a traditional risk factor for CKD.

For each identified patient, there are 0.51 undiagnosed conditionally ill individuals with the same non-traditional risk factors for CKD. The detectability of non-traditional risk factors per patient is from 3.40 to 4.58 risk factors, respectively.

3.2. The significance of microalbuminuria/ proteinuria as a predictor of diagnosis and risk factor for the development of chronic kidney disease

The main diagnostic method for CKD is a urine test, where proteinuria and changes in urine sediment are detected. But these changes are usually detected in stages 4-5 of CKD, when specific clinical symptoms of kidney damage appear. In the asymptomatic current stages of CKD and in the absence of clinically obvious proteinuria, a urine test for microalbuminuria allows diagnosis in the early stages of chronic kidney damage.

A reliable value of proteinuria is the determination of its amount on the daily urine of the subjects, which is more than

0.5 g per day, which usually corresponds to a MAU of ≤ 300 mg per day.

The determination of proteinuria in daily urine requires special conditions for the collection of urine. Currently, a system of test strips for urine analysis is widely used in the clinical laboratory, which simultaneously contain the ability to determine microalbumin and creatinine in the urine of the examined individuals.

To clarify the probability of MAU, the albumin/creatinine ratio (ACR) was determined. This ratio was evaluated on the following scale: Normal - normal; Abnormal - pathology; Highabnormal-pronounced pathology.

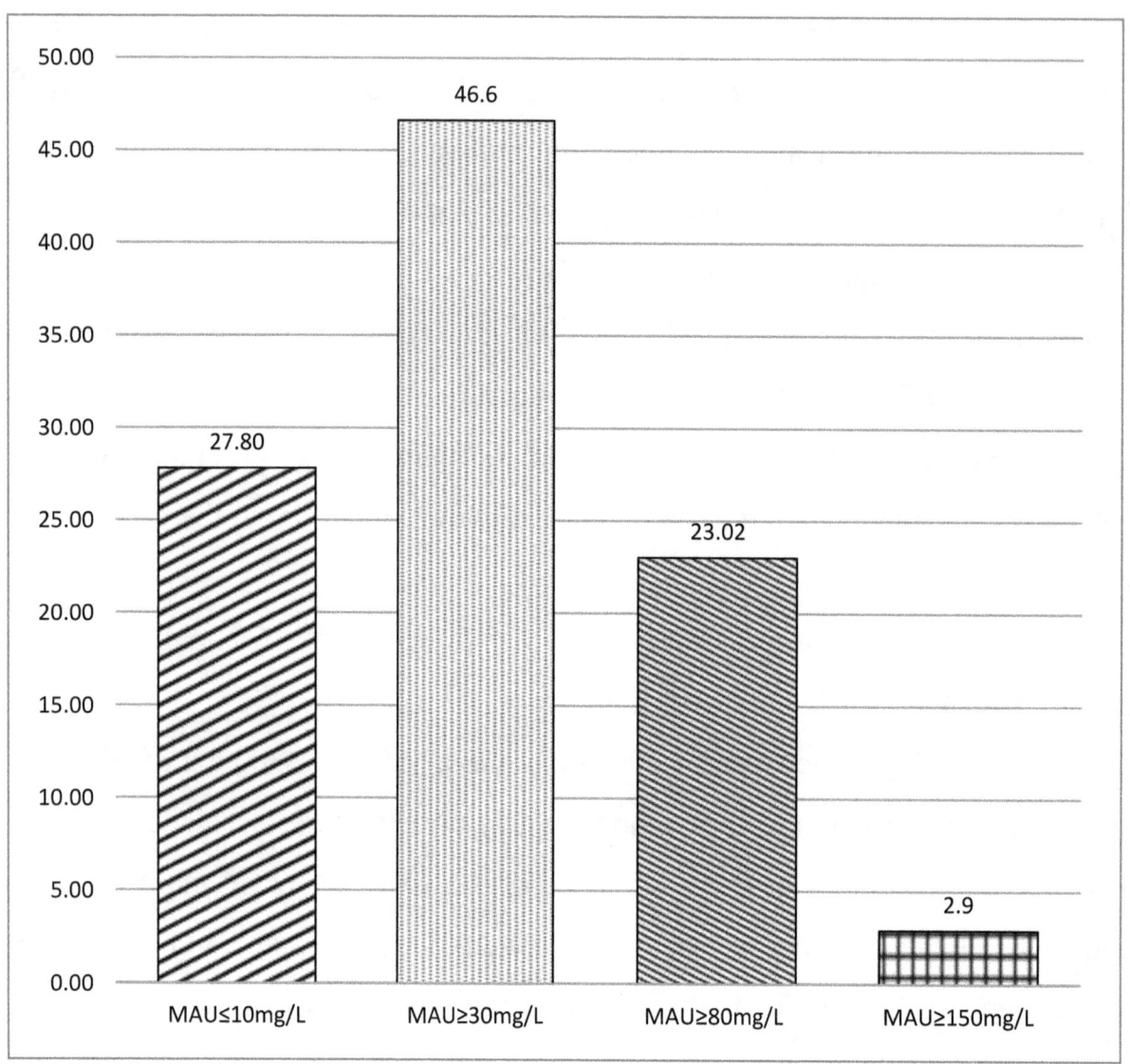

3. 1. The prevalence of albuminuria in the examined patients, depending on the degree of MAU (in %)

The initial increase in microalbuminuria (MAU=10-30 mg/l) was determined in 46.33±4.98% (n=40), the average increase (30-80 mg/l) in 23.03±4.20% (n=20)and the high level of MAU (80-150 mg/l) in 2.84±1.66% (n=2) cases. (Fig. 3. 1.)

Studies have shown that there is a direct proportional relationship between the frequency of CKD risk factors and a certain level of microalbuminuria (Figure 3.2).

It was found that with an increase in the level of UIA, the detection of risk factors also increases. This proven relationship is especially noticeable when studying such a risk factor as arterial hypertension: 18.64±3.64% with MAU=10-30 mg/l;

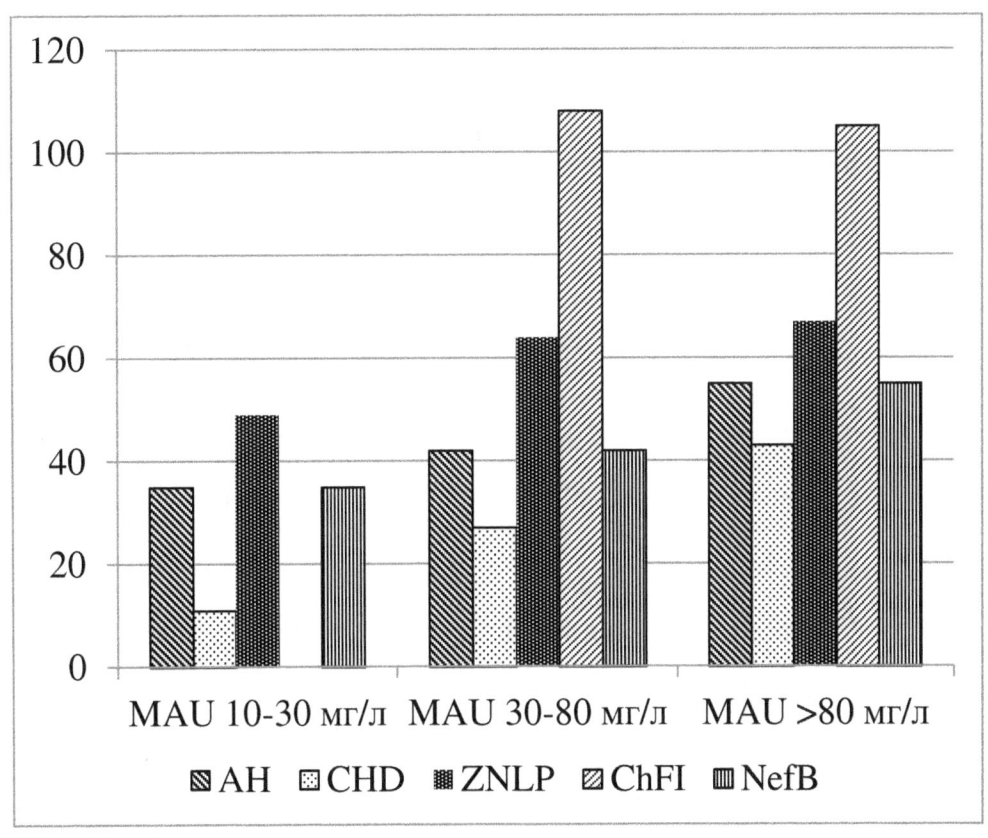

37.74±4.84% with MAU=30-80mg/l and 43.62±4.95% with MAU>80mg/l; in addition, the same picture was observed with the incidence of coronary heart disease: 13.75±3.43% with MAU=10-30 mg/l; 32.51±4.68% with MAU=30-80mg/l and 53.75% with±4.98% at MAU>80mg/l. The same data were obtained for the risk factor of abuse of nephrotoxic drugs 21.78±4.37% for MAU=10-30 mg/l, 33.68±4.72% for MAU=30-80mg/l and 35.26±4.77% for MAU>80mg/l; Similar indicators were obtained for the presence of chronic foci of infection with the following indicators: 21.78±4.37% for MAU=10-30 mg/l; 33.68±4.72% for MAU=30-80mg/l and 35.26±4.77% at MAU>80mg/l. It is especially necessary to mention such a risk factor as, nephropathy of pregnant women in the anamnesis in women, where the following parameters were obtained: 26.51±4.41% with MAU=10-30

Figure 3.2. Frequency of occurrence of risk factors in the examined patients depending on the level of microalbuminuria

Note: MAU – microalbuminuria; AH - arterial hypertension; CHD – ischemic heart disease; ZNLP-abuse of nephrotoxic drugs; NKHOI – the presence of chronic foci of infection; NefB b A- nephropathy of pregnant women in the anamnesis.

In the examined patients, whose MAU level is within the normal range (MAU= 10 mg / l), but a pathological deviation of the creatinine/microalbumin ratio (ACR-abnormal) is determined, the frequency of detection by a risk factor for CKD development showed the following parameters:

- arterial hypertension in 18.64±3.64% (n=16) cases;
- coronary heart disease in 13.75±3.43% (n=10) cases;
- abuse of nephrotoxic drugs in 25.87±4.37% (n=22) cases;
- the presence of chronic foci of infection in 18.38±3.87% (n=16) cases;
- a history of nephropathy in pregnant women in 26.51±4.41% (n=23) cases

.It is known that albuminuria is used as an early marker of glomerular filter damage, but in proteinuria and / or MAU, the renal tubules are also damaged at the same time. Proteins that enter the primary urine have a toxic effect on the cells of the tubular epithelium and activate the development of tubulointerstitial fibrosis [Nats. recom.CKD, RF 2012].

To determine the value of MAU as a risk factor for the development and / or progression of CKD, we analyzed the relationship between the level of microalbuminuria and the stage of CKD (Figure 3.3.).

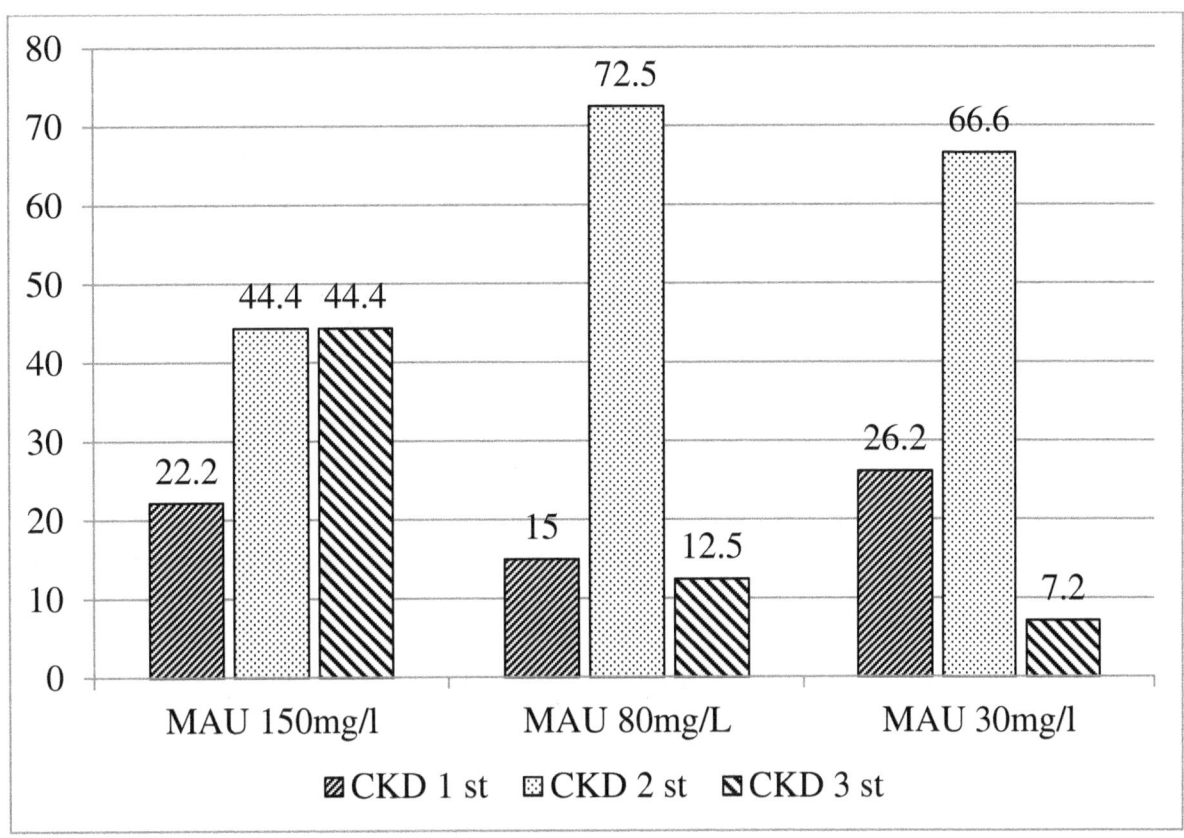

Figure 3.3. Prevalence of microalbuminuria depending on the stage of CKD in the examined patients

Among the examined persons (n=87) with an established diagnosis of CKD, 28.7±4.52% were found. The distribution of MAU by CKD stages was as follows: with an initial increase in MAU (30 mg / l), the occurrence of stage 3 CKD was in 7.14±2.57% of cases, stage 2 in 66.66±4.71% and stage 1 in 26.19±4.39% of cases (p<0.001).

Among the examined population with an increase in the level of MAU to 80 mg / l, the incidence of stage 3 CKD was 12.5±3.3%; stage 2 72.5±4.96% and stage 1 15.0±3.5% (p<0.01); with a level of MAU greater than 150 mg/l, stage 3 CKD was found in 38.9±4.87%, stage 2 38.9±4.87%; stage 1 CKD in 22.22±4.15% (p<0.01) of the examined patients.

Thus, the definition of MAU has diagnostic value and allows earlier identification of patients of different risk groups with CKD. The determination of MAU on an outpatient basis will allow for early diagnosis of CKD, in addition, this method will allow for effective primary and secondary prevention. Microalbuminuria, which is a predictor of early diagnosis of CKD, is also a risk factor for CKD. An increase in the level of proteinuria / microalbuminuria worsens the prognosis of CKD. Given the close, direct relationship between the amount of albumin excreted in the urine and the degree of CKD development, it can be concluded that MAU is particularly important in the development and progression of CKD in the examined patients.

From the above, we can conclude that the early detection of UIA in screening examinations has several features:

- first, microalbumin is an early diagnostic predictor, when it is detected in the urine, which is 8-10 years earlier will allow the diagnosis of CKD before the manifestation of specific clinical symptoms of kidney damage in addition, in this sense, MAU is of great importance as a prognostic risk factor for CKD, cardiovascular pathologies and diabetes mellitus;
- second, early detection of UIA will allow to determine CKD in the initial stages, which improves the quality of life of patients and reduces the cost of RRT in ESRD;
- Third, the definition of UIA allows for secondary prevention of CKD and reduces the likelihood of CKD progression.

§ 3.3. The algorithm optimizes the tactics of early detection of chronic kidney disease and ways to prevent progression.

Effective policies for the prevention of chronic kidney disease rely on indicators of the incidence and prevalence of this disease, as well as on the frequency of distribution and the burden of risk factors for development.

The most modern method of identifying the prevalence of risk factors and the significance of their effect on the development of CKD is screening.

Screening is a purposefully organized secondary prevention measure to detect the disease at the preclinical stages and the main goal is to detect the disease earlier before the onset of clinical symptoms. Under screening.also understand the mass survey of the population from a certain risk group or "conditionally healthy" who do not go to doctors. At the same time, the goal of screening is to reduce morbidity, disability and death from their complications.

- Based on the conducted scientific research, we propose the following measures of primary and secondary prevention of CKD:

Conducting a screening survey of the population to identify risk factors and determine the risk group for CKD (including the age from 18 to over 45 years.

Taking into account the difficulties and inexpediency of continuous screening of the population for the detection of CKD, as well as the high cost and labor intensity of laboratory tests during mass surveys among the population (representatives of the conditionally healthy population and the active working population), the first place is proposed to conduct a questionnaire to identify prognostically significant risk factors for chronic kidney disease.

At the same time, people who fill out the questionnaire are informed about the causes of development and clinical symptoms of CKD. This provides two-way benefits: first, increasing the medical education of the population, and second, they try to create a healthy lifestyle based on this information.

- Create an electronic register of the population at risk of developing CKD;
- Given the diagnostic value of microalbuminuria for the early detection of CKD, it is advisable to determine this parameter for the diagnosis of CKD once a year in people at risk on an outpatient basis;
- Create an information sheet in outpatient records that contains complete information about non-traditional CKD risk factors (body mass index, OT, OB, bad habits, information about frequently used medications, the presence of chronic foci of infection, about diseases of direct line relatives that are an unfavorable risk factor for CKD) and systematically updates this data to determine the effectiveness of prevention and/or treatment measures;
- Repeated blood and urine tests with the determination of creatinine and urea, calculation of GFR, microalbumin in the urine in women with nephropathy and hypertension during pregnancy, 1 time per year;
- Appropriate planning of consultations with nephrologists 1 and / or 2 times a year (based on the degree of the risk group Annex 2) for the population at

risk for the timely and effective detection and treatment of CKD in the early stages.

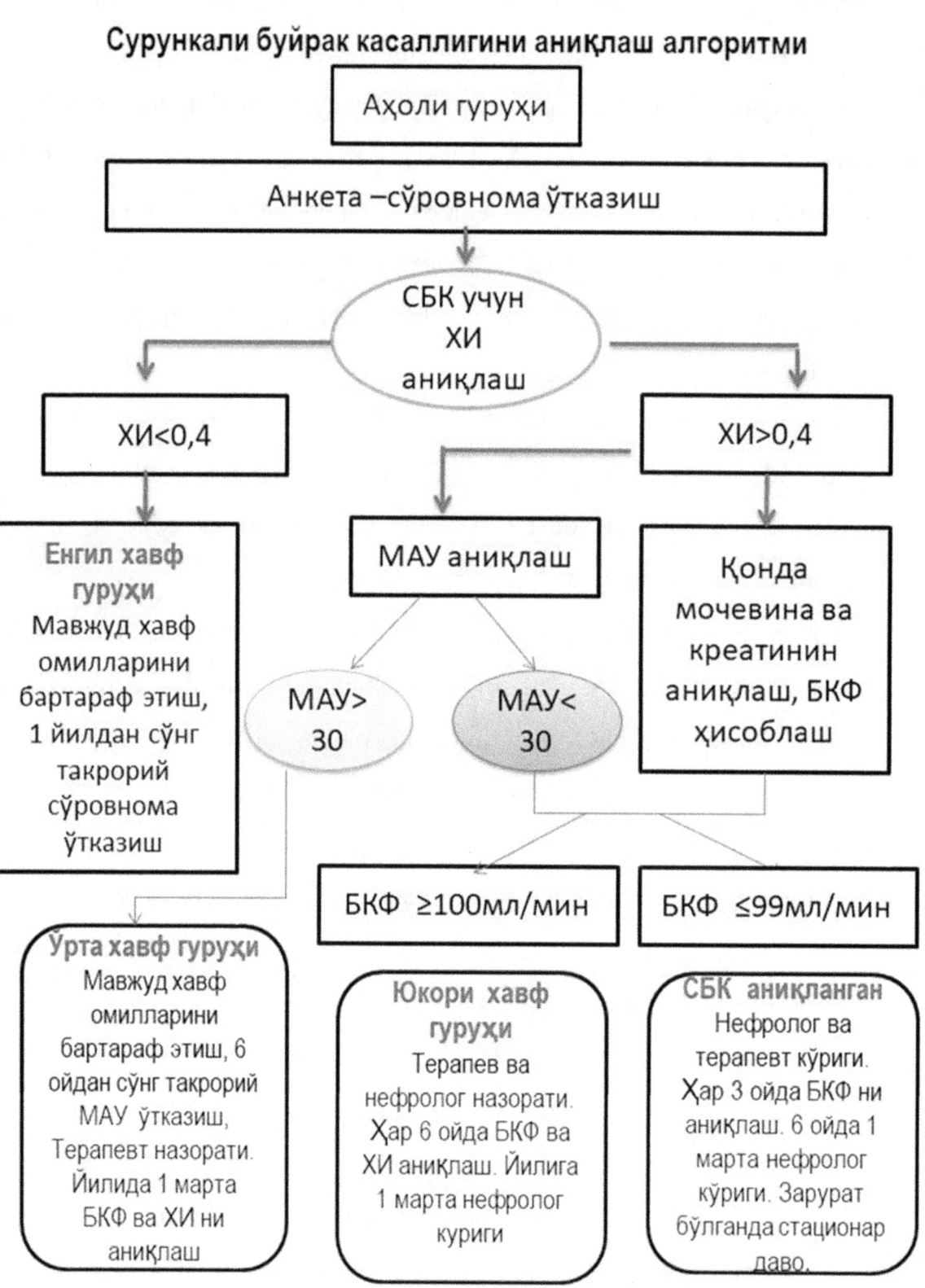

SUMMARY

Numerous clinical and socio-medical studies conducted in the world over the past decades provide a complete picture of the scale of CKD problems that have spread to all countries of the world. The prevalence of CKD is high and is not inferior to the prevalence of such socially significant diseases as diabetes mellitus, hypertension, and heart failure

The literature data of recent years show that the prevalence of CKD and its range varies from 10-18%. This is due to the different criteria that are used for screening for CKD, as well as the place of residence (city or village), ethnic customs, lifestyle and standard of living, the effectiveness of preventive measures, the spread of chronic non-communicable diseases among the population.

In our study, we raised the question of determining the prevalence of chronic kidney disease at its various stages in the population..

Developed national and international recommendations from different countries offer a number of markers for the early diagnosis of CKD. With a decrease in GFR of 60 ml / min, the functional and structural damage to the kidneys will undoubtedly be irreversible, however, it is possible to identify earlier-reversible-stages, which should first be paid attention to.

To date, the study of albuminuria is of paramount importance for the early diagnosis of CKD, when there is no proteinuria and a decrease in GFR, as well as for assessing the risk of its progression and the development of complications – both in the early and later stages. The simplicity and accessibility of this method of diagnosing CKD is an important advantage that is necessary for conducting screening studies.

In our studies, the diagnosis of CKD was established in accordance with international recommendations and the available diagnostic capabilities of each treatment and prevention institution.

A microalbuminuria test and GFR calculation using the CKD-EPI formula for creatinine and MDRD were performed in the health care unit. When comparing these two GFR markers, the advantages of either of them were not revealed, which makes it possible to use them interchangeably.

Until recently, serum creatinine concentrations were considered to be the main estimates of GFR in practical medicine all over the world.

The introduction of these two methods in the diagnostic standards at the primary health care level (in outpatient settings) increases the chance of early diagnosis of the development and progression of CKD.

Our data on the prevalence of chronic kidney disease in certain population groups suggest that its occurrence in general is not lower than in the world. According to our data, the prevalence of CKD among women of the active working population was 28.7%. The distribution by stages of CKD was as follows: 1 st. - 12.6%, 2 st. - 13.2%, 3 st. - 2.8%. The high prevalence of stages 1 and 2 was associated with a high frequency of risk factors: arterial hypertension, overweight, obesity, the presence of chronic foci of infection, abuse of nephrotoxic drugs.nephropathy of pregnant women in the anamnesis in women.

In outpatient settings, where it is not possible to study daily urine, we examined the level of albumin in a single portion of urine in patients using test strips. The criterion for CKD was AU ≥ 30 mg/l. As a result, high albuminuria was detected in 29.2% of the examined patients.

The results of our study showed that the questionnaire plays an important role in identifying risk factors for chronic kidney disease.

In our study, the division of the questionnaire into blocks containing complaints characteristic of CKD, nephrological history data, indications of metabolic disorders and family predisposition to them, information about maintaining a healthy lifestyle allows us to more accurately identify risk factors for CKD and determine indications for laboratory examination, which is important both for improving the detection of CKD, especially in its early stages, and for the rational appointment of laboratory tests.

The second set of questions in the questionnaire concerned the presence of patient complaints. The most specific complaints were those directly related to kidney damage and uremia, such as dysuria, nocturia, pain and discomfort in the lower back. However, their sensitivity to the risk of MAU ≥ 30 mg/L was relatively low. The most sensitive predictors were complaints such as swelling of the limbs and eyelids. Complaints of edema, which can be observed both in independent kidney disease and in cardiovascular pathology, are characterized by a combination of high sensitivity and specificity.

Among the representatives of the conditionally healthy population, there was a difference in complaints in different sex and age groups. In younger people, there were complaints of edema, and among women of this age, pain in the lower back, dysuria with nocturia. The older age group was characterized by thirst and dysuria. The most common risk factors for CKD in our study were arterial hypertension, overweight, obesity, the presence of chronic foci of infection, and the abuse of nephrotoxic drugs.

Attention is drawn to the revealed association of high MAU with the presence of nephropathy in women with a history of pregnancy.

We found a significant association of high albuminuria with the abuse of analgesics. Frequent use of analgesics poses an immediate threat to the kidneys, since these drugs can have a toxic effect on the epithelium of the renal tubules, and also contribute to their ischemic damage by suppressing the production of prostaglandins.

In our studies, it was noticeable that there is a large difference in the indicators of kidney changes according to ultrasound studies, the frequency of MAU ≥ 30 mg/l in the examined patients is significantly higher than certain pathological changes in the kidneys during ultrasound.

To date, the place of ultrasound in the diagnosis of CKD remains not fully defined. Population studies for the detection of CKD were based on laboratory data – the determination of GFR and MAU, but, as a rule, did not include ultrasound data.

In our studies, only anamnesis data was taken into account and does not give an idea of what specific symptoms of structural changes in the kidneys during ultrasound were observed in the examined patients.

It seems important that by filling out the questionnaire and passing a subsequent interview with a doctor, the subject gets an idea of the factors that adversely affect the kidneys, he develops a more conscious attitude to the need to lead a healthy lifestyle in order to prevent CKD and an understanding of the need for regular preventive medical examinations. These questionnaires allow not only to assess the risk of CKD, but also to create an individual program of nephroprophylaxis and nephroprotection, taking into account the characteristics of the patient's condition.

CONCLUSIONS

1. The prevalence of CKD in women of childbearing age increased with age. The level of diagnosis of CKD as a nosological unit is quite low. Among the examined patients, who were diagnosed on the basis of outpatient records, the diagnosis of CKD as a nosological unit was not revealed. After the examination, this diagnosis was established in 29.1% (n=21) of the respondents from the general subjects.

2. Using questionnaires in population groups, risk factors for the development of CKD were identified, which were related to traditional ones, such as arterial hypertension, cardiovascular pathology, diabetes mellitus, as well as non-traditional factors such as nephropathy of pregnant women in the anamnesis in women, overweight, abuse of nephrotoxic drugs, the presence of foci of chronic infection in the body, hyperlipedemia, which have an independent significance in the development of CKD.

3. Microalbumin is an early diagnostic predictor, when detected in the urine, which is 8-10 years earlier will allow the diagnosis of CKD before the manifestation of specific clinical symptoms of kidney damage. In addition, in this sense, MAU is of great importance as a prognostic risk factor for CKD.

4. The algorithm for detecting CKD in women of fertile age allows using a questionnaire to select from the initial population of patients with high risk for subsequent examination of laboratory markers (serum creatinine and albuminuria) for the final diagnosis of CKD.

PRACTICAL RECOMMENDATIONS

1. To identify chronic kidney disease among women of fertile age, at the first stage, a questionnaire is recommended (according to aspecially designed questionnaire) in order to identify individuals with a high risk of developing CKD.
2. In the future, among this group, a study of laboratory markers is conducted: microalbuminuria, serum creatinine with the calculation of GFR and, depending on the result, CKD is diagnosed.
3. For primary and secondary prevention of the development and progression of CKD, it is important to introduce the definition of microalbuminuria in outpatient settings, as a predictor of the diagnosis of CKD.
4. For the early diagnosis of CKD among women of childbearing age who are at risk and with massive screening examinations that do not involve blood tests, it is possible to detect CKD with the help of an albuminuria study.

СПИСОК ЛИТЕРАТУРЫ

1. Авдеева М.В., Шкодина Н.В. Патология почек и риск развития сердечно-сосудистых заболеваний. Бюллетень ВСНЦ со РАМН. 2011 №1. Часть 1 стр 28-29
2. Агранович Н.В. «Обоснование и эффективность профилактики и лечения больных с хронической болезнью почек в амбулаторно-поликлинических условиях» Нефрология. 2013. Том 17. №5.
3. Александрова, Ирина Игоревна. Ранняя диагностика нарушений нутритивного статуса у больных хронической почечной недостаточностью, факторы риска их развития. : диссертация ... кандидата медицинских наук : 14.01.29 / Александрова Ирина Игоревна; [Место защиты: ГОУВПО "Московская медицинская академия"].- Москва, 2013.- 82 с.
4. Алферов С.М., Дурникин М.А. Спектр возбудителей при различных формах пиелонефрита // Тезисы III Всероссийской научно-практической конференции с международным участием «Рациональная фармакотерапия в урологии- 2014». Москва. С.9.
5. Антонова Т.Н., Бикбов Б.Т., Галь И.Г., Томилина Н.А. К вопросу о распространенности хронической болезни почек среди пожилых лиц в г. Москве и ее связи с сердечно-сосудистой патологией // Нефрол. и диализ. 2011. N23. С.353-354.
6. Ахмедова Н.Ш., Абдуллаев Р.Б. Значение определения микроальбуминурии как предиктор диагностики хронической болезни почек//«Тиббиётнинг долзарб муаммолари» Ёш олимлар XXV илмий-назарий анжумани материаллари. – Урганч, 2018 С. 452-453
7. Ахмедова Н.Ш. Фертил ёшдаги аёлларда сурункали буйрак касалликлари учраш сабаблари ва унинг профилактикаси // Она ва бола саломатлигини муҳофаза қилишнинг долзарб муаммолари, ютуқлари ва истиқболлари Республика илмий-амалий анжумани материаллари.– Бухоро, 2018. С. 154
8. Ахмедова Н.Ш. Оценка факторов риска, ассоциированнх с альбуминурией,

вляющих на развитие хронический болезни почек // International Scientific and Practical CONFERENCE Trends in Science and Technology.– Warsaw, Poland, 2018. Vol.2, P 24-27

9. Ахмедова Н.Ш. Особенности скрининга почечной функции в амбулаторных условиях // MEDICUS (International medical journal). –Волгоград, 2019, № 2(26). – С 17-21

10. Бестаева Т. Л. 11. Влияние минерально-костных нарушений на развитие сердечно-сосудистых осложнений при хронической болезни почек. Автореф .дис. на соиск. учен. степ. канд. мед. наук Владикав каз, 2015. 22, [1] с.

11. Бикбов Б. Т. Раннее выявление хронической болезни почек: маркер преемственности в лечении пациентов, влияние на выживаемость и кардиоваскулярную летальность больных на диализе. // Российский медицин-ский журнал. 2014 (№ 1. 2014 С. 11-17.

12. Бова А.А. Хроническая болезнь почек как независимый фактор риска сердечно-сосудистой патологии. Ж. К помощи к военному врачу. С.П. Т1. .01.2014 г стр 15-20

13. Бородулин В.Б., Протопопов А.А., Горемыкин В.И. Диагностика хронической болезни почек в ранней стадии //Клиническая нефрология. 2014. №2.С.52-55.

14. Васильева М. П. Цистатин С - новый маркер гипертрофии миокарда левого желудочка у пациентов с хронической болезнью почек. // Терапевтический архив. 2015 (Т. 87, № 6. 2015 С. 17-22.

15. Васильева И.А., Добронравов В.А., Панина И.Ю., Трофименко И.И., «Качество жизни больных на различных стадиях хронической болезни почек» Нефрология. 2013. Том 17. №2.

16. Вельков В.В. NGAL - «ренальный тропонин», ранний маркер острого повреждения почек: актуальность для нефрологии и кардиохирургии. Клинико-лабораторный консилиум 2011; 38(2): 90-100

17. Вялкова А.А, Лебедева Е.Н и др. Клинико –патогенетические аспекты повреждения почек при ожирение. Нефрология. 2014. Том 18. №3.

18. Гажонова В. Е. Прогностическое значение индекса резистентности сосудов почек в оценке прогрессирования хронической болезни почек.// Терапевтический архив. 2015 (Т. 87, № 6. 2015 С. 29-33.

19. Галушкин А.А., Батюшин М.М., Терентьев В.П., Горблянский Ю.Ю. «Комплексная оценка сердечно-сосудистых факторов риска, как инструмент прогнозирования развития хронической болезни почек» Нефрология. 2013. Том 17. №5.

20. Горностаева Е.Ю. Влияние вегетативной нервной системы на развитие хронической болезни почек у больных метаболическим синдромом : автореферат дис.. кандидата медицинских наук - Москва, 2010 - 25 с.

21. Давыдкин И.Л., Шутов А.М., Ромашева Е.П. Анемия при хронической болезни почек: руководство / М.: ГЭОТАР-Медиа, 2013. 64 с.

22. Деревянченко М.В. Особенности функционального состояния почек и показателей метаболизма у больных артериальной гипертензией, обусловленной хроническим пиелонефритом // IV Национальный конгресс терапевтов (XX Съезд российских терапевтов). Сборник материалов. Москва, 2009. С. 77.

23. Джуманова Р.Г., Турусбекова А.К., Калиев Р.Р. Влияние дисфункции эндотелия на почечную гемодинамику у больных с хроническими заболеваниями печени Clinical medicine of Kazakhstan, volume 1, number 31 (supplement 1 (2014)) научно-практический медицинский журнал

24. Дзгоева Ф. У. 23-й фактор роста фибробластов и новый высоко-чувствительный тропонин I: ранние маркеры и альтернативные пути поражения сердца при хронической болезни почек. // Терапевтический архив. 2015 (Т. 87, № 6. 2015 С. 68-74.

25. Дзгоева Ф. У. Остеопротегерин и 23-й фактор роста фибробластов (FGF-23) в развитии сердечно-сосудистых осложнений при хронической болезни почек. // Терапевтический архив. 2014 (Т. 86, № 6. 2014 С. 63-69.

26. Добронравов В.А., Богданова Е.О., Семенова Н.Ю. Цинзерлинг В.А., Смирнов А.В. «Почечная экспрессия белка aklotho, фактор роста

фибробластов 23 и паратиреоидный гормон при экспериментальном моделировании ранних стадий хронического повреждения почек» Нефрология. 2014. Том 18. №2.

27. Жидкова Т. Ю. К характеристике эндотелиальной дисфункции и структурно-функционального состояния левых камер сердца у пациентов с артериальной гипертонией и хроническим пиелонефритом: автореф. дисс. канд. мед. наук. Екатеринбург, 2010. 32 с.

28. Земченков А.Ю., Герасимчук Р.Л., Костылева Т.Г., Виноградова Л. Ю., Земченкова И.Г. Книга для пациентов на диализе «Жизнь с хроническим заболеванием почек» //. СПб., 2011.

29. Камышлов В.С. Методы клинических лабораторных исследований. ООО «МЕДпресс-информ», 2013. 736 с.

30. Карпачева Н.А., Петросян Э.К. Возможности ранней диагностики хронической болезни почек у подростков при диспансеризации //Клиническая нефрология. 2013. №1. С.44-48.

31. Каюков И.Г., Смирнов А.В., Эмануэль ВЛ. Цистатин С в современной медицине. Нефрология 2012; 16 (1): 22-39

32. Клинические практические рекомендации по Хроническому Заболеванию Почек: Оценка, Классификация и Стратификация. URL: http://www.dialysis.ru/standard/doqi-ckd/g7.htm (дата обращения - 2012 г.).

33. Ковелина О.С. Хронические болезни почек в сочетании с другими заболеваниями внутренних органов и их факторами риска : диссертация кандидата медицинских наук Челябинск, 2008.- 156 с.

34. Кузнецова Т. Е. Вариабельность синусового ритма сердца у больных хронической сердечной не достаточностью с признаками хронической болезни почек. Дис. на соиск. учен. степ. канд. мед. наук Нижний Новгород, 2015. 148 с.

35. Кузьмин О.Б. Механизмы развития и прогрессирования нефропатии у больных сердечной недостаточностью с хроническим кардиоренальным синдромом. Нефрология 2011;15, 2:20-29

36. Курапова, М.В. Изменение микроциркуляторного русла при хронической болезни почек / Актуальные вопросы полиморбидной патологии в клинике внутренних болезней: сборник тезисов 5-й Международной научно-практической конференции.- Белгород, 2013. - С. 67-68.

37. Кутырина И. М. Факторы риска поражения сердечно-сосудистой системы при хронической болезни почек. // Терапевтический архив. 2013 (Т. 85, № 9. 2013 С. 69-76.

38. Лукичёв Б. Г. Современное состояние вопроса об использовании энтеросорбции при хронической болезни почек. // Нефрология. 2014 (Т. 18, № 6. 2014 С. 43-50.

39. Лукичёв Б.Г., Подгаецкая О.Ю., Карунная А.В., Румянцев А.Ш. «Индоксил сульфат при хронической болезни почек» Нефрология. 2014. Том 18. №1

40. Милованова Л. Ю. . Роль морфогенетических белков FGF-23, Klotho и гликопротеина склеростина в оценке риска развития сердечно-сосудистых заболеваний и прогноза хронической болезни почек. // Терапевтический архив. 2015 (Т. 87, № 6. 2015 С. 10-16.

41. Мирончук Н. Н. Функциональное состояние почек и система гемостаза у больных с хронической сердечной недостаточностью ишемического генеза. Автореф .дис. на со- иск. учен. степ. канд. мед. наук Челябинск, 2014.24 с.

42. Мухин Н. А.Диагностика и лечение болезней почек: руководство. М.: ГЭОТАР-Медиа, 2011. 384 с.

43. Нагайцева С. С., Швецов М.Ю., Герасимов А.Н. и др. «Исследование альбуминурии как маркера хронической болезни почек у взрослого трудоспособного населения» Альманах клинической медицины № 30 '2014

44. Нагайцева С.С. Факторы риска повышения альбуминурии как раннего маркера хронической болезни и почек в разных возрастных групп пах.// Нефрология. 2013 (Т. 17, № 4. 2013 С. 58-62.

45. Нагайцева С.С., . Швецов М.Ю, Шалягин Ю.Д., Пягай Н.Л., Шилов Е.М. «Факторы риска повышения альбуминурии как раннего маркера хронической болезни почек в разных возрастных группах» Нефрология.

2013. Том 17. №4.

46. Нагайцева С.С., Швецов М.Ю., Герасимов А.Н. и др. Статификация риска развития хронической болезни почек с помощью анкетирования //Клиническая нефрология. 2014. №1.С.15-23.

47. Нагайцева С.С., Швецов М.Ю., Шалягин Ю.Д. и др. Оценка альбуминурии методом тест-полосок с целью раннего выявления хронической болезни почек у лиц с разной степенью риска (опыт Центров здоровья Московской области) // Тер. арх. 2013. N26. С.38-43.

48. Национальные рекомендации. Сердечно-сосудистый риск и хроническая болезнь почек: стратегии кардио-нефропротекции. 2013. 55 с.

49. Национальные рекомендации. Хроническая болезнь почек: основные принципы скрининга, диагностики, профилактики и подходы к лечению //Клиническая нефрология. 2012. № 4. С. 4-26.

50. Нефрология /под ред. Е. М. Шилова. М.: ГЭОТАР-Медиа, 2007. С. 599612.

51. Нефрология. Ключи к трудному диагнозу / М.М. Батюшин. ЗАО НПП «Джанагар», 2007. С.168.

52. Никитина А.О. Управление формированием интегративных санаторно-курортных комплексов в регионе. Монография. Санкт П. 2012 г. 290 ст

53. Николаев А.Ю., Милованов Ю.С. Лечение почечной недостаточности: руководство для врачей. М: Медицинское информационное агентство, 2011. С. 592.

54. Павлова И. В. диссертация на теме «Клинико- лабораторные и функциональные проявления мочевого синдрома у пациентов с хронической болезнью почек. методы коррекции» 2015 г

55. Пелевин А.Р. Функциональное состояние почек у больных с метаболическим синдромом. Возможности медикаментозной коррекции: автореферат дис. . кандидата медицинских наук : Тюмень, 2012 - 19 с.

56. Похильченко М. В. Хроническая болезнь почек у пациентов с артериальной гипертензией 1-2 степени молодого возраста : автореферат дис. ... кандидата медицинских наук : Москва, 2015 - 22 с.

57. Пролетов Я.Ю., Саганова Е.С., Галкина О.В., Зубина И.М., Богданова Е.О. «Роль некоторых биомаркеров в оценке характера хронического повреждения почек у пациентов с первичными гломерулопатиями » Нефрология. 2013. Том 17. №1

58. Рафрафи Т.Н. Величина скорости клубочковой фильтрации как фактор ремоделирования сердца на ранних стадиях хронической болезни почек. Автореферат диссертации на соискание ученой степени кандидата медицинских наук. Санкт-Петербург 2011. 34 стр

59. Рафрафи Т.Н., Дегтерева О. А., Каюков И.Г., Добронравов В.А., Никогосян Ю.А., Куколева Л.Н. Смирнов А.В. К проблеме оценки величины скорости клубочковой фильтрации у пациентов с хронической болезнью почек// Нефрология. -2011. - Т. 15, №1. - С. 104-110.

60. Руденко Л. И. Прогнозирование риска развития сердечно-сосудистой кальцификации у пациентов с хронической болезнью почек, получающих заместительную почечную терапию гемодиализом. Автореф .дис. на соиск. учен. степ. канд. мед. наук Ростов-на-Дону, 2015. 24 с. :

61. Сивков А.В., Синюхин В.Н., Бебешко Е.В. Уремический токсин паракрезол у больных с терминальной стадией ХПН. Экспериментальная и клиническая урология 2012; №1: 68-71

62. Abdel-Kader K, Greer RC, Boulware LE, Unruh ML: Primary care physicians' familiarity, beliefs, and perceived barriers to practice guidelines in non-diabetic CKD: a survey study. BMC Nephrol 15: 64, 2014

63. Adamczak M, Wiecek A: The adipose tissue as an endocrine organ. Semin Nephrol 33: 2-13, 2013

64. Akbari A, Clase CM, Acott P, Battistella M, Bello A, Feltmate P, Grill A, Karsanji M, Komenda P, Madore F, Manns BJ, Mahdavi S, Mustafa RA, Smyth A, Welcher ES: Canadian Society of Nephrology Commentary on the KDIGO Clinical Practice Guideline for CKD Evaluation and Management. Am J Kidney Dis 65: 177-205, 2015

65. Alberti KG, Zimmet P, Shaw J: Metabolic syndrome—a new world-wide

definition. A Consensus Statement from the International Diabetes Federation. DiabetMed23: 469-480, 2006

66. Alexander RT, Hemmelgarn BR, Wiebe N, Bello A, Morgan C, Samuel S, Klarenbach SW, Curhan GC, Tonelli M;Alberta Kidney Disease Network: Kidney stones and kidney function loss: A cohort study. BMJ 345: e5287, 2012

67. American College of Physicians. Screening, Monitoring, and Treatment of Stage 1 to 3 Chronic Kidney Disease: A Clinical Practice Guideline From the American College of Physicians // Annals of Internal Medicine. 2013. Vol. 159(12). P. 835-847.

68. Appleton SL, Seaborn CJ, Visvanathan R, Hill CL, Gill TK, Taylor AW, Adams RJ; North West Adelaide Health Study Team: Di¬abetes and cardiovascular disease outcomes in the metabolically healthy obese phenotype: A cohort study. Diabetes Care 36: 2388-2394, 2013

69. ArnlovJ, Ingelsson E, Sundstram J, Lind L: Impact of body mass index and the metabolic syndrome on the risk of cardiovascular disease and death in middle-aged men. Circulation 121: 230¬236, 2010

70. Arora P, Vasa P, Brenner D, Iglar K, McFarlane P, Morrison H, Badawi A: Prevalence estimates of chronic kidney disease in Canada: results of a nationally representative survey. CMAJ 185: E417-E423, 2013

71. Asian Pacific Society of Nephrology. Assessment of kidney function in type 2 diabetes // Nephrology. 2010. Vol. 15. P.146-161.

72. Assogba GF, Couchoud C, Roudier C, Pornet C, Fosse S, Romon I, Druet C, Stengel B, Fagot-Campagna A: Prevalence, screening and treatment of chronic kidney disease in people with type 2 diabetes in France: the ENTRED surveys (2001 and 2007). Diabetes Metab 38: 558-566, 2012

73. Claudia M. Lora, Lisa Nessel, Ana C. Ricardo, Julie Wright Nunes, Michael J. Fischer, and the CRIC Study Investigators Predictors and Outcomes of Health-Related Quality of Life in Adults with CKD Clin J Am Soc Nephrol 11: 1154-1162, July, 2016

74. Desai AS, Toto R, Jarolim P, Uno H, EckardtK-U, Kewalramani R, Levey AS,

Lewis EF, McMurray JJV, Parving H-H, Solomon SD, Pfeffer MA: Association between cardiac biomarkers and the development of ESRD in patients with type 2 diabetes mellitus, anemia, and CKD. Am J Kidney Dis 58: 717-728, 2011